AF436071

The ADHD Toolkit -

Strategies for thriving in a fast-paced world

Author Oak Erkul
Editor and illustrator Harlund Leaf

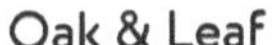

Oak & Leaf

Acknowledgments

We would like to extend our sincerest thanks to all the individuals with ADHD who have shared their experiences and contributed to this book.

Your insights and perspectives have been invaluable in helping to educate and inform the world about ADHD.

We also thank our family, friends, and colleagues for their support and encouragement throughout the writing process. Without their love and encouragement, this book would not have been possible.

Finally, we would like to acknowledge the hard work and dedication of the healthcare professionals, researchers, and advocacy organizations who work tirelessly to improve the lives of individuals with ADHD.

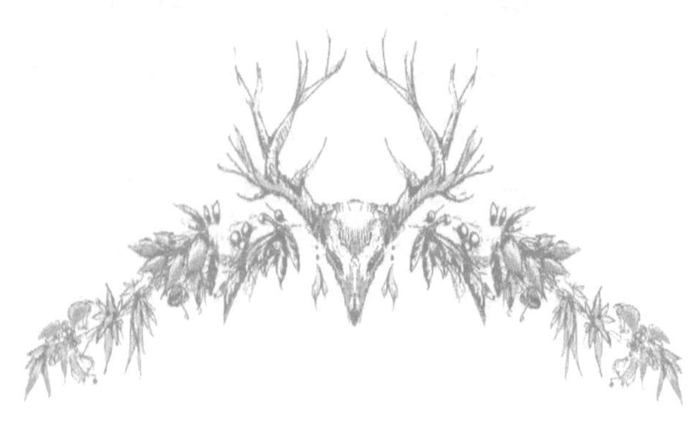

"The only limit to our realization of tomorrow will be our doubts today."

- Franklin D. Roosevelt

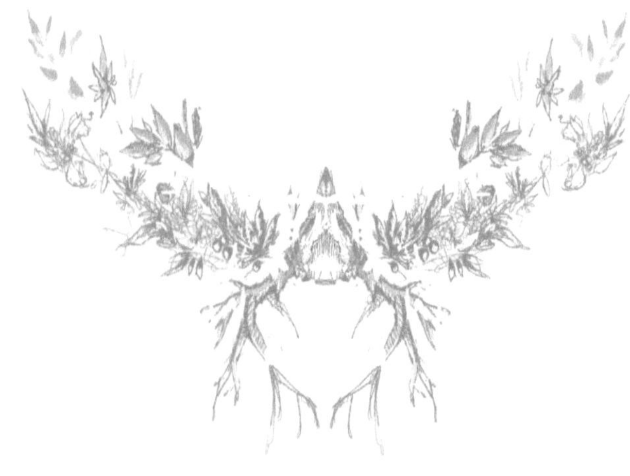

Content

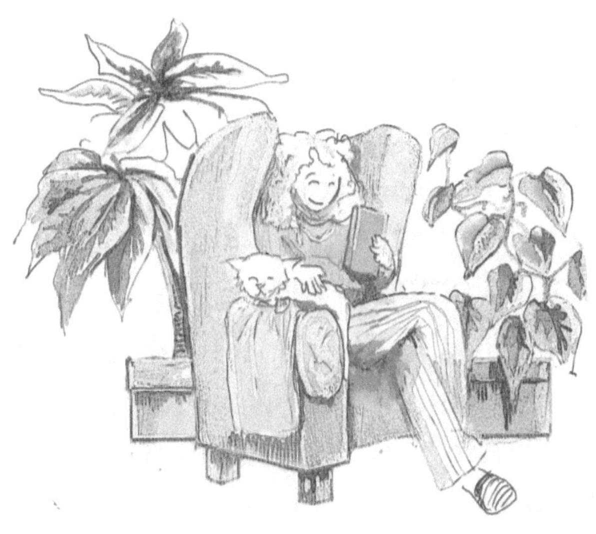

If you're reading this, chances are you or someone you care about is living with ADHD, and you're looking for ways to manage the challenges and make the most of your life. We're here to help.

Living with ADHD can be tough. The symptoms of ADHD, such as impulsivity, inattention, and difficulty with organization and time management, can make daily life feel overwhelming at times. But it's important to remember that you are not alone.

Millions of people around the world live with ADHD, and there are effective strategies and treatments available to help manage the disorder. This book is designed to provide you with the tools and resources you need to take control of your ADHD and improve your quality of life.

We'll cover a range of topics, including time management, self-care, relationships, and education and employment.

Whether you're looking for tips on how to organize your schedule or ways to cope with the challenges of ADHD, you'll find something here that can help.

We encourage you to read through the book at your own pace and to try out the strategies that resonate with you. Remember, there's no one-size-fits-all solution to managing ADHD, and what works for one person may not work for others.

Beginning of the Journey

Working on oneself can be a challenging and rewarding process, and this is especially true for individuals with ADHD.

ADHD is a neurodevelopmental disorder that affects attention, impulsivity, and hyperactivity. It can often lead to difficulties with time management, organization, and self-regulation, which can make it difficult to make progress in various areas of life.

However, with the right strategies and support, people with ADHD can work on themselves and make meaningful progress towards their goals.

On the next couple of pages we've written an overview of some steps that can help people with ADHD to begin working on themselves, or atleast have an idea of where to start.

Afterwards we'll go a bit more in depth on each subject, so as to get a better feel for how to go about working with yourself

Overview

Seek a proper diagnosis

The first step in addressing ADHD is to seek a proper diagnosis from a healthcare provider.

This can help to confirm that ADHD is the cause of any difficulties you may be experiencing, and will allow you to develop a treatment plan that is tailored to your specific needs.

Learn about ADHD

Once you have received a diagnosis of ADHD, it can be helpful to learn as much as you can about the disorder.

Understanding how ADHD affects you and what strategies may be helpful in managing your symptoms can be empowering and can help you feel more in control of your life.

Find a support system

Having a strong support system of friends, family, and other loved ones can be very beneficial when working on oneself.

A support system can provide encouragement, motivation, and a sense of belonging, which will be helpful in the journey towards self-improvement.

While not everyone have a Support system, remember that you can build one without having to have family and friends, but

instead try to engage in group therapy either online or in person. Here you can support each other and get a feel for the fact that you are not alone with your struggles.

Identify your goals

It's a good idea to identify specific goals that you want to work towards. These could be related to your career, relationships, health, or personal growth.

Once you have identified your goals, you can begin to develop a plan for achieving them.

Seek professional help (besides getting the diagnosis)

Working with a mental health professional, such as a therapist or counselor, can be a valuable part of the process of working on oneself.

A therapist can help you to identify and address any underlying issues that may be contributing to your difficulties and can provide support and guidance as you work towards your goals.

Use strategies to manage your ADHD

There are many strategies that can be helpful in managing the symptoms of ADHD.

These may include medication, therapy, mindfulness practices, exercise, proper rest and natural remedies.

While we will go over different ways to use tools and strategies for self-help in this book, remember that some might resonate well with you where others might not be the most appropriate for your individual needs.

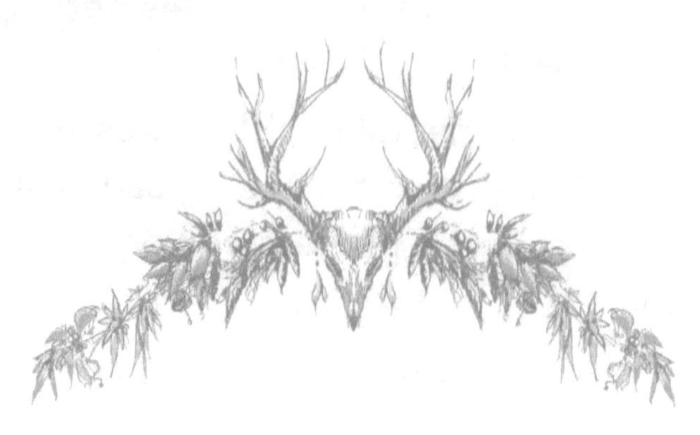

"We are what we repeatedly do.
Excellence, then, is not an act, but a habit."

- Aristotle

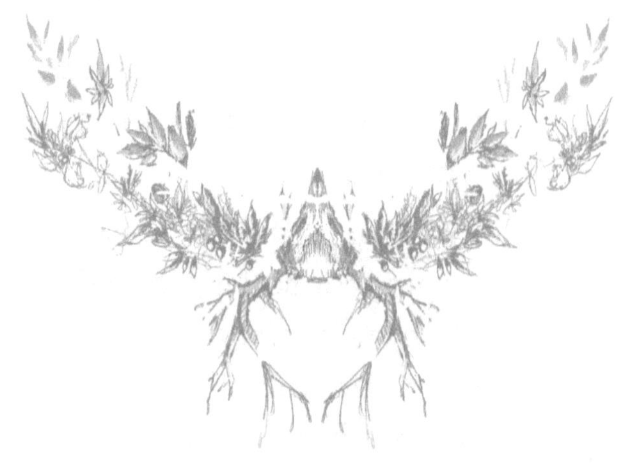

Seeking a proper diagnosis

First and foremost, a proper diagnosis can help you understand your own symptoms and behaviors.

Knowing that you have ADHD can help you make sense of challenges you have faced in the past and may be facing currently. It can also provide a sense of relief, as it can be validating to know that there is a reason for the difficulties you have experienced and that you are not alone in your struggles. A proper diagnosis can also provide you with access to appropriate treatment options.

While there is no cure for ADHD, there are a number of effective treatments that can help you manage your symptoms and improve your overall functioning. These treatments may include medication, therapy, proper dieting and rest, or most likely- a combination of all of them.

A healthcare professional can help you determine the most appropriate treatment plan for your needs. Additionally, a proper diagnosis can help you better advocate for yourself in various settings, such as at work or in school.

Having a diagnosis can provide access to accommodations that can help you be more successful in these settings. For example, in some situations you may be able to request extra time on exams or have a designated quiet space to work in.

If you are in need of medication to better handle your symptoms in your daily life, a proper diagnosis will also help you focus on which kind of medication will have the best effect on your individual needs with the least amount of side effects.

Learning about ADHD

First a bunch of facts about ADHD

Attention-deficit/hyperactivity disorder (ADHD) is a neurodevelopmental disorder that affects an estimated 5% of children and 2.5% of adults worldwide.

It is characterized by difficulty with attention, impulsivity, and hyperactivity.

These symptoms can cause significant challenges in daily life, including problems with school or work performance, relationships, and self-regulation.

One of the most significant ways that ADHD affects people is by interfering with their ability to focus and pay attention.

People with ADHD may have trouble focusing on tasks, following instructions, or completing projects. This can lead to problems with school or work performance, as they may have difficulty paying attention in class or meetings, or may make careless mistakes.

Impulsivity is another common symptom of ADHD. People with ADHD may have trouble controlling their impulses, leading to problems with decision-making and self-regulation. They may act on their impulses without thinking about the consequences, which can lead to problems with relationships, finances, and safety.

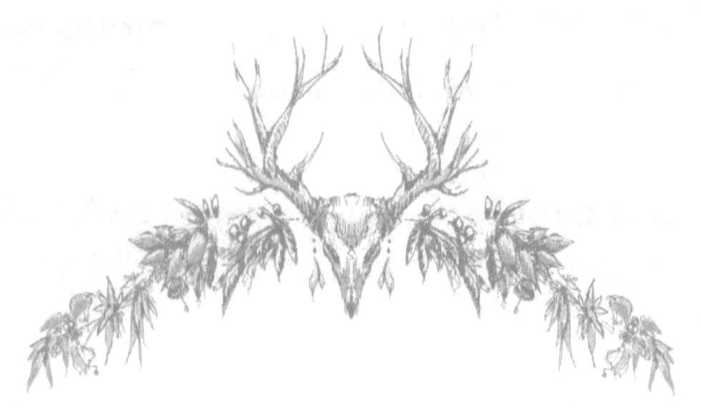

"*Hardships often prepare ordinary people for an extraordinary destiny.*"

C.S. Lewis

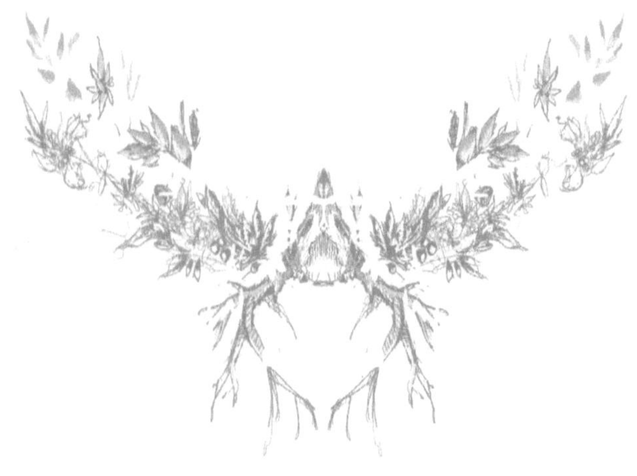

Hyperactivity is another symptom of ADHD that can have a significant impact on daily life. People with ADHD may have difficulty sitting still or may feel constantly restless. This can lead to problems in school or work, as they may have difficulty remaining seated or may struggle to complete tasks that require prolonged periods of focus.

In addition to these core symptoms, people with ADHD may also struggle with executive function skills such as organization, planning, and time management. This can make it difficult to manage their daily lives, leading to problems with clutter, punctuality, and meeting deadlines.

The challenges associated with ADHD can have a significant impact on a person's overall well-being. People with ADHD may struggle with low self-esteem, anxiety, and depression. They may also have problems with relationships, as their impulsivity and difficulty with focus and attention can lead to misunderstandings and conflict with others.

However, it is important to note that ADHD is a somewhat treatable disorder, even though there's no actual "cure". With proper dieting, rest and self-care exercises you can get far, and with the help of a healthcare provider you can develop a plan that's tailored to your individual needs.

Support System

Having a strong support system can be incredibly beneficial for people with ADHD, as it can provide encouragement, motivation, and a sense of belonging.

A support system can also help to alleviate feelings of isolation, which can be common among people with ADHD.

While not everyone has close family or friends that they can rely on, there are alternatives such as groups with similar issues, self-help teams and coaches.

Here are some steps that you can take to find a support system

Identify your needs

Start by identifying what you need from a support system. This might include emotional support, practical help, or someone to talk to about your experiences with ADHD.

Reach out to loved ones

A good place to start when looking for a support system is with friends and family. These are people who know you well and are likely to be supportive and understanding. You might consider talking to a close friend or family member about your experiences with ADHD and asking for their support.

Join a support group

Another option is to join a support group for people with ADHD. Support groups can be a great way to connect with others who are dealing with similar challenges. You can find ADHD support groups through local hospitals, mental health clinics, or online resources.

Consider therapy

Therapy can be a helpful tool for building a support system, as it provides a safe and confidential space to discuss your thoughts and feelings with a mental health professional. A therapist can provide support and guidance as you work through challenges related to ADHD.

Seek out online resources

There are many online resources available for people with ADHD, including forums, blogs, and social media groups. These can be a great way to connect with others who are dealing with similar challenges and to find support and guidance.

Consider finding an ADHD coach

ADHD coaching is a specialized form of coaching that focuses on helping people with ADHD to develop strategies for managing their symptoms and achieving their goals. An ADHD coach can provide support and guidance as you work on building a support system and improving your overall well-being.

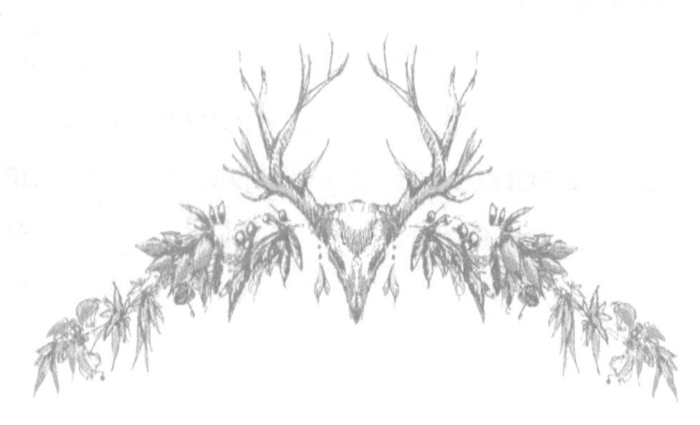

"*Life is 10% what happens to us and 90% how we react to it.*"

\- Charles R. Swindoll

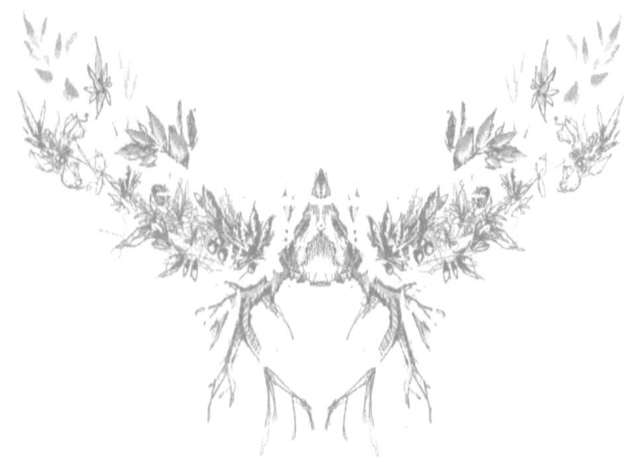

Identify your goals

Identifying goals can be a powerful tool for people with ADHD, as it helps to provide focus and direction and can be motivating. However, it can also be challenging for people with ADHD to set and achieve goals, as the symptoms of the disorder can interfere with focus, organization, and self-regulation.

Start small

It can be overwhelming to try to tackle too many goals at once, especially for people with ADHD. It can be helpful to start with small, achievable goals and to build up to larger ones over time.

Break goals down into smaller steps

Large goals can be intimidating, and it can be helpful to break them down into smaller, more manageable steps. This can help to make progress feel more attainable and can help to keep you motivated.

Set specific and measurable goals

Vague or unspecific goals can be difficult to work towards, as it can be hard to know when you have achieved them. It can be helpful to set specific and measurable goals, such as "I will study for one hour each day" or "I will run a 5k race within the next three months." This will help you to know when you have achieved your goal and to track your progress.

Identify any obstacles

Try to identify any obstacles that may get in the way of achieving your goals. This might include challenges related to your ADHD, such as difficulty with focus or organization. By identifying these obstacles ahead of time, you can develop strategies for overcoming them.

Use time-management techniques

As it is easy to lose track of time and get disorientated with your daily life, it's a good idea to find different time-management techniques that work for you. We will be going

over a few later in this book, but basically
you need some way to keep a track of what's
important and when it needs to be done.

Be patient

Achieving goals can take time, and it is important to be patient and to celebrate your progress along the way. Don't get discouraged if you don't achieve your goals as quickly as you had hoped – focus on the progress you have made and keep working towards your goals.

By following these steps, people with ADHD can identify and work towards their goals in a way that is manageable and sustainable. Remember that achieving goals takes time and effort, but the sense of accomplishment and progress that comes with it can be incredibly rewarding.

Professional Help

While ADHD can be managed effectively with proper treatment, many people with ADHD do not seek professional help.

There are several reasons why it is advisable that you seek professional help. Professional help can improve the quality of life for individuals with ADHD.

Professional help can also address comorbid conditions that often occur with ADHD. These may include anxiety, depression, and substance abuse. By treating these conditions, you can better manage their overall mental health.

There are several options for seeking professional help. Psychotherapy, such as cognitive-behavioral therapy, can help you with learning coping strategies and change negative patterns of thinking and behavior.

Medication, such as stimulants or non-stimulants, can also be effective in managing ADHD symptoms.

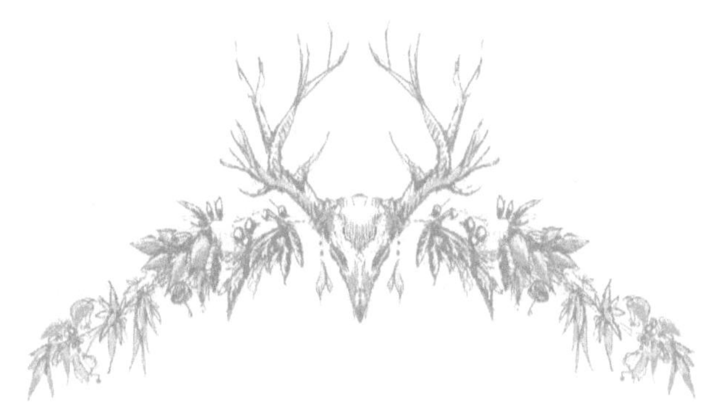

"It's not about having
the strength to go on; It's about
finding the strength to start over."

-unknown

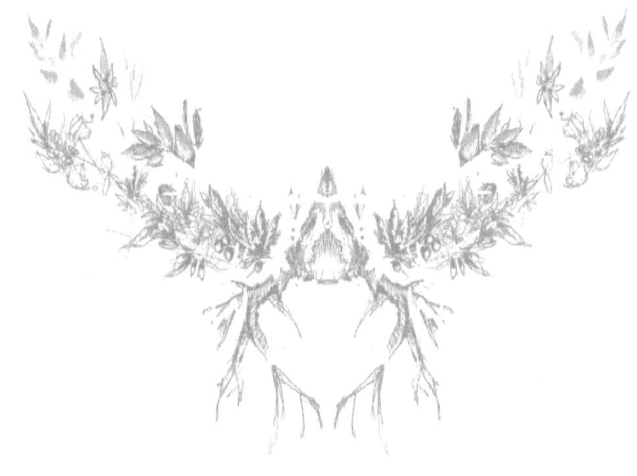

Strategies to manage your ADHD

Managing ADHD can be challenging, but luckily there's a number of strategies that you can use to better manage their symptoms and improve their overall quality of life.

Lifestyle changes

Making changes to your daily routine and environment can also be helpful in managing ADHD. This may include setting aside dedicated times for focusing on tasks, breaking large tasks into smaller ones, and creating a structured and organized

environment. It may also be helpful to limit distractions and find ways to relax and unwind.

Medication

Stimulant medications, such as Ritalin and Adderall, are often used to treat ADHD. These medications can help improve focus and attention, as well as reduce impulsivity. It is important to work closely with a healthcare professional to determine the best medication and dosage for your needs.

Therapy

As mentioned earlier, therapy is an important factor that many skip all together. There's therapy such as cognitive behavioral therapy (CBT), which can help individuals with ADHD learn coping strategies for managing their symptoms. A therapist can work with you to identify negative thought patterns and behaviors and teach you new ways of thinking and acting.

Parenting strategies

For parents of children with ADHD, learning positive parenting strategies can be helpful in managing their child's behavior. This may include setting clear expectations, giving consistent consequences for inappropriate behavior, and providing positive reinforcement for good behavior. It may also be helpful to work with your child's school to develop a plan for managing their ADHD in the classroom.

Children with ADHD may benefit from accommodations in the classroom, such as extra time on tests or assignments, or the use of assistive technology. It is important to work with your child's school to determine what accommodations would be most helpful.

Self-Care strategies

Self-Care is actually the most important factor, and there's many individual parts of Self-Care that can help you quite a bit with managing your symptoms and overall life.

Here's some of the more important ones

Exercise

Exercise has been shown to have a number of benefits for individuals with ADHD. Physical activity can improve focus and concentration, as well as reduce stress and improve mood. It can also help with impulse control and increase self-esteem. It is recommended that adults get at least 150 minutes of moderate-intensity aerobic activity, such as brisk walking, or 75 minutes of vigorous-intensity activity, such as running, each week. Children and adolescents should get at least 60 minutes of moderate- to vigorous-intensity physical activity each day.

Sleep and Taking Breaks

Getting enough quality sleep is essential for managing ADHD. Lack of sleep can exacerbate symptoms such as impulsivity and inattention. To improve sleep quality, it is recommended to establish a regular sleep routine, create a relaxing bedtime routine, and avoid screens and other stimuli before bedtime. It is also important to create a comfortable sleep environment, such as keeping the bedroom cool, dark, and quiet.

Taking breaks and allowing oneself time to rest and recharge is necessary for managing ADHD. This may involve setting aside dedicated relaxation time, or taking short breaks throughout the day to do something enjoyable. It is also important to listen to one's body and pay attention to signs of burnout or overwhelm.

Proper diet

A healthy diet can have a positive impact on focus and concentration, as well as overall physical and mental health. It is recommended to eat a diet that is rich in fruits, vegetables, and protein, and to limit or eliminate processed foods and sugary drinks. Some studies have also suggested that certain nutrients, such as omega-3 fatty acids, may be helpful in managing ADHD symptoms.

Time management

Time management is another issue you might be having trouble with. It's Very common for people with ADHD to have problems with Time, which is why there's quite a few very useful tools for exactly that. In the next chapter we'll go over a few different techniques and in the back there's gonna be quite a few blank tool pages you can use in your daily life.

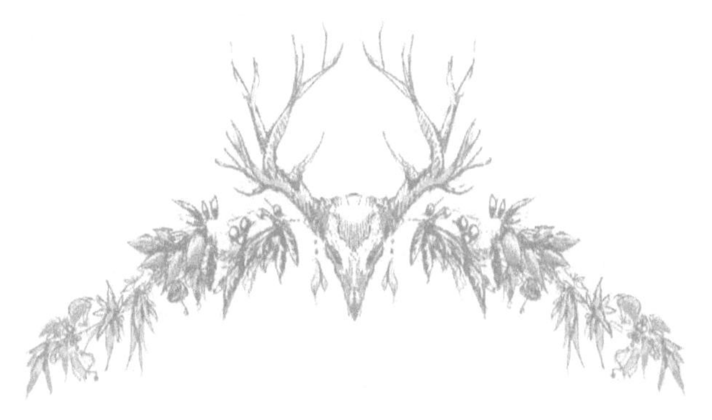

"Don't watch the clock; do what it does.
Keep going."

-Sam Levenson

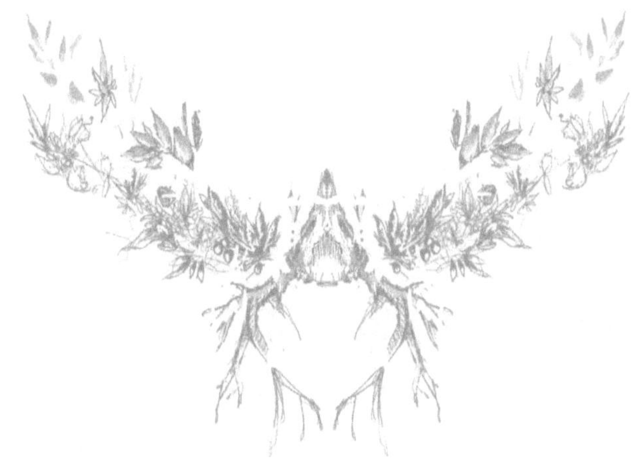

ADHD in the Workplace

Communicate with your employer

Try to be open and honest with your employer about your ADHD. They may be able to provide accommodations or support that can help you be successful in your role.

Use time management techniques

Time management can be a challenge for individuals with ADHD, but there are a number of strategies that can help. These may include using a planner or calendar to keep track of tasks and appointments, breaking large tasks into smaller ones, and setting aside dedicated times for focusing on tasks. It may also be helpful to limit distractions and find ways to relax and unwind.

Consider medication

Medicine isn't always the best choice as it does come with some side effect, but it's worth considering in some workplaces as it does help with focus and overall concentration.

Stimulant medications, such as Ritalin and Adderall, are often used to treat ADHD and can help improve focus and attention. Please work closely with a healthcare professional to determine the best medication and dosage for your needs if you do want to use medication.

Take breaks

It is important to take breaks throughout the workday to rest and recharge. This can help improve focus and productivity. Consider setting aside a few minutes each hour to stretch, take a walk, or engage in a relaxing activity.

Use assistive technology

Assistive technology, such as text-to-speech software or a planner app, can be helpful for individuals with ADHD. These tools can help with organization, task management, and communication.

Find a job that fits your strengths

People with ADHD often have unique strengths and abilities that can be valuable in the workplace. Consider looking for a job that aligns with your strengths and interests.

Try to stay positive

It can be easy to get discouraged when living with ADHD, but it's important to stay positive and focus on your successes.

Remember to celebrate your accomplishments and take pride in the progress you've made.

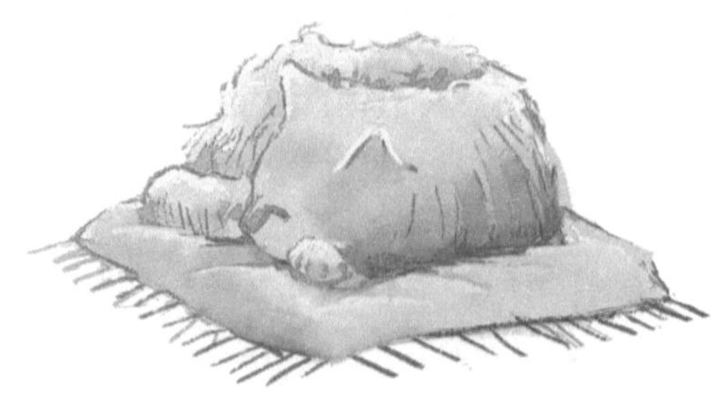

Time Management Techniques

The Eisenhower Box

The Eisenhower Box, also known as the Eisenhower Matrix, is a time management tool that can be useful for individuals with ADHD or anyone looking to prioritize tasks and manage their time more effectively. The Eisenhower Box helps individuals to identify which tasks are urgent and important, and which tasks are less urgent or important. This can be helpful in managing ADHD because it allows individuals to focus on the most important tasks first, rather than becoming overwhelmed by a long to-do list.

A Instead of thinking about it, do this now
B Schedule this for a designated time period later
C Things that needs to be done, but not necessarily by you
D No need to waste energy, just delete this

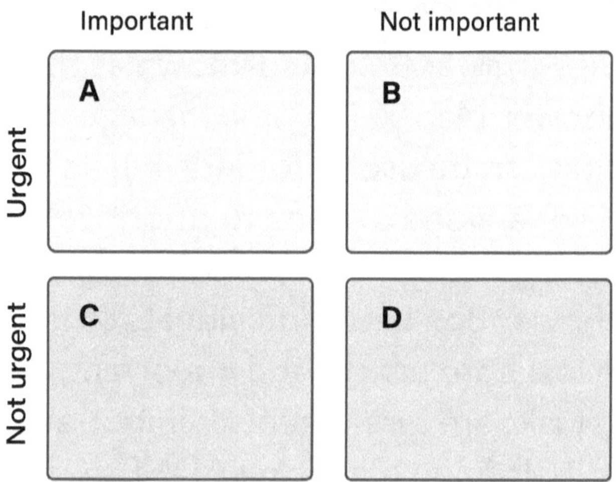

To use the Eisenhower Box, you will need to

Draw a simple grid with four quadrants.

Label the top row "Urgent" and the bottom row "Not Urgent.", Label the left column "Important" and the right column "Not Important."

List your tasks in one of the four quadrants based on their level of urgency and importance.

Spend the majority of your time working on

tasks in the "Important" and "Urgent" quadrants. These are the tasks that require your
immediate attention.

The task in the "Not Important" and "Urgent"
quadrant is something you need to have
done soon, but it's not your main priority at
this time- Schedule a designated time in your
calendar to do this later.

Consider delegating tasks in the "Important"
and "Not Urgent" quadrants to others to free
up more time for the important tasks.

The Pomodoro Technique

The Pomodoro Technique is a time management method developed by Francesco Cirillo in the late 1980s. It involves working in focused, 25-minute intervals (called "pomodoros") followed by a short break. This can be helpful for individuals with ADHD because it allows for frequent breaks, which can help maintain focus and prevent burnout.

To use the Pomodoro Technique, follow these steps:

Choose a task to work on.

Set a timer for 25 minutes (or any other interval that works for you).

Work on the task until the timer goes off.

Take a short break (usually 5-10 minutes).

Repeat the process for a total of four pomodoros

Take a longer break (30-45 min) before you repeat the process. (if you aren't done with the project)

The ABC Method

The ABC Method is a technique for prioritizing tasks on your to-do list.

This method is a lot like the Eisenhower box, but here you can write it directly in your calendar or planner. The Eisenhower box gives a better overall overview of the tasks, but the ABC method is faster to use.

To use this method, follow these steps

Make a list of all the tasks you need to complete.

Assign a priority level to each task, "A" for tasks that are important and urgent, "B" for tasks that are important but not urgent, and "C" for tasks that are not important.

Work on the "A" tasks first, followed by the "B" tasks, and then the "C" tasks.

Consider delegating or eliminating "C" tasks if possible.

The "Two-Minute Rule"

The "Two-Minute Rule" is a simple but effective time management technique that can help you avoid procrastination and stay on top of small tasks. The idea behind the rule is that if a task can be completed in two minutes or less, it should be done immediately. This can help prevent small tasks from becoming overwhelming and prevent them from getting lost in a long to-do list.

Here's how the "Two-Minute Rule" works

Make a list of all the tasks you need to complete.

Go through the list and identify any tasks that can be completed in two minutes or less. These might include tasks like sending an email, filing a piece of paper, or making a phone call.

Do these tasks immediately. Don't put them off or save them for later.

For tasks that take longer, break them down into smaller, more manageable steps. For example, if you need to write a report, you might break the task down into smaller steps like research, outline, write draft, and revise.

By following the "Two-Minute Rule," you can stay on top of small tasks and prevent them from becoming overwhelming. This can help improve your productivity and reduce stress.

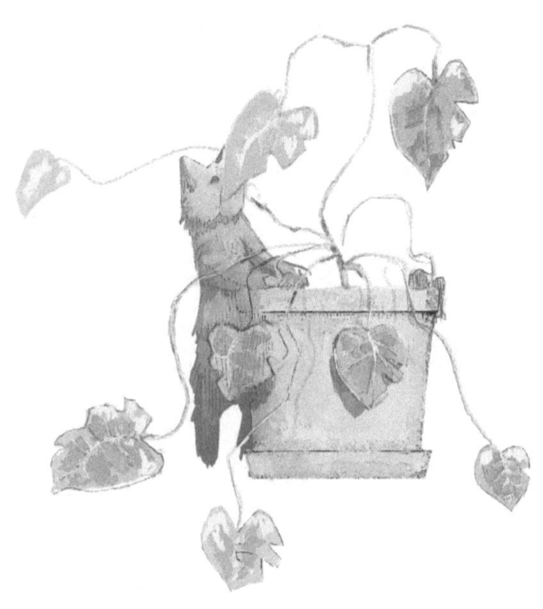

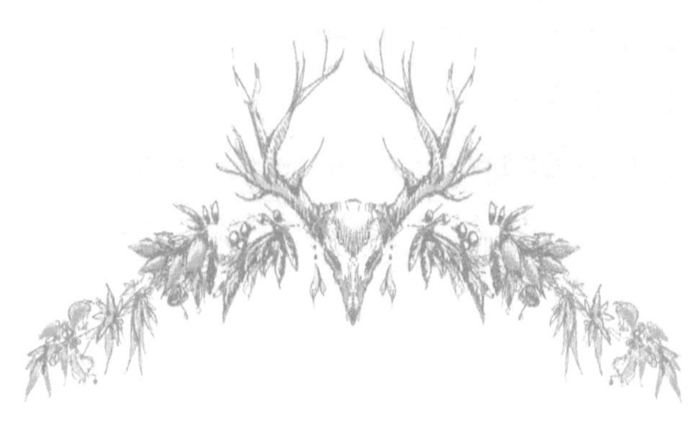

"Believe you can and you're
halfway there."

- Theodore Roosevelt

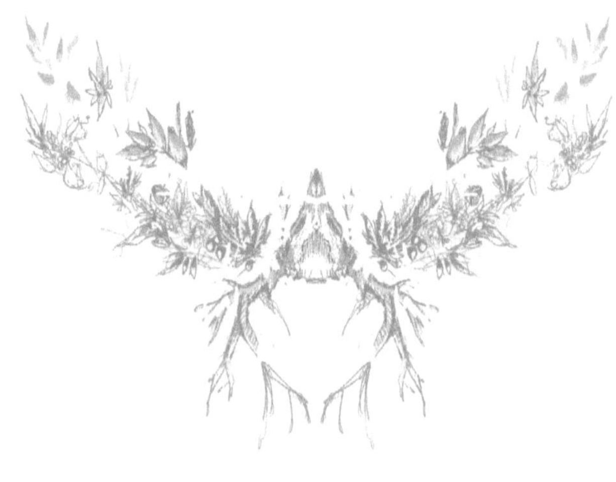

Meditation Techniques

Mindfulness Meditation

Mindfulness meditation is a simple, yet powerful practice that involves bringing one's attention to the present moment in a non-judgmental way. It is a form of meditation that can be practiced by anyone, anywhere, at any time, and has been shown to have numerous physical, mental, and emotional benefits.

The practice of mindfulness involves paying attention to our thoughts and feelings in the present moment, without trying to change them or judge them. It involves cultivating a sense of curiosity and openness towards one's own experience, and developing the ability to let go of distractions and focus on the present moment. This can be done by paying attention to one's breath, the sensations in one's body, or the sounds and sights around us.

One of the main benefits of mindfulness meditation is the reduction of stress and anxiety. When we are mindful, we are better able to recognize and acknowledge our thoughts and emotions, rather than getting lost in them or reacting automatically to them. This can help us to respond to difficult situations in a more mindful and considered way, rather than reacting impulsively or becoming over-whelmed by our emotions.

Mindfulness meditation can also improve focus and concentration. By regularly practicing mindfulness, we can train our minds to be more present and less prone to distraction. This can be especially useful in today's fast-paced world, where our attention is often pulled in multiple directions at once.

In addition to these mental benefits, mindfulness meditation has been shown to have physical benefits as well. It has been linked to a range of positive health

outcomes, including lower blood pressure, improved immune function, and reduced chronic pain.

Mindfulness meditation can also have positive effects on our relationships and sense of well-being. By being more present and attuned to our own thoughts and feelings, we can become more aware of the needs and emotions of others, and develop greater empathy and understanding. This can lead to deeper, more fulfilling relationships with others.

Overall, mindfulness meditation is a powerful practice that can bring numerous benefits to our lives. Whether we are dealing with stress and anxiety, struggling to focus, or simply seeking a greater sense of well-being, mindfulness meditation can be a valuable tool to help us find greater peace and contentment in our lives.

To start Mindfulness Meditation

Find a quiet and comfortable place to sit or lie down. You can use a meditation cushion or sit on a chair with your feet planted firmly on the ground. It's important to find a position that allows you to be comfortable and alert.

Close your eyes and take a few deep breaths, focusing on the sensation of the breath as it enters and leaves your body. This can help to ground you in the present moment and bring your attention inward.

Bring your attention to the present moment by focusing on your senses. Notice what you see, hear, smell, taste, and feel in the present moment. You can focus on one sense at a time, or scan through all of your senses. The goal is to cultivate a sense of curiosity and openness towards your experience.

When your mind wanders (which it will), gently redirect your attention back to your senses in the present moment. It's natural for the mind to wander, and this is not a sign of failure. Simply notice when your mind has wandered, and gently bring your attention back to the present moment.

Continue this process for 10-20 minutes, or for as long as you like. You can use a timer to keep track of the time, or simply focus on your breath and let the time pass.

**Prompts you can use during the meditati-
on**

"I am present."

"I am aware of my breath."

"I am aware of my senses."

"I am aware of my thoughts, but I am not my
thoughts."

"I let go of my thoughts and return to the
present moment."

Meditation is a practice, and it may take
some time and effort to get the hang of it.
Be patient with yourself and try not to get
discouraged if your mind wanders or you
have difficulty focusing. Just keep coming
back to the present moment and your breath,
and over time, you will begin to see the benefits of meditation in your daily life.

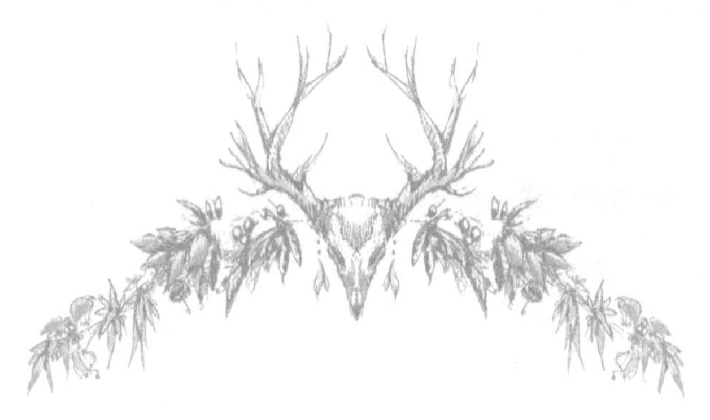

"Happiness is not something ready-made.
It comes from your own actions."

-Dalai Lama

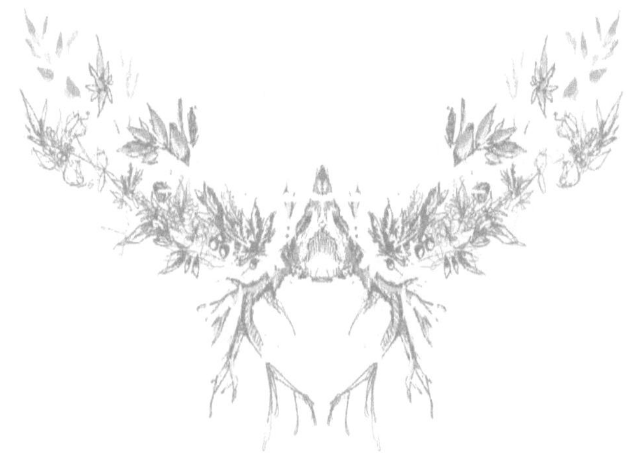

Body scan meditation

Body Scan is a technique that involves lying down and focusing on the sensation of each part of the body, starting at the toes and moving up to the top of the head. It is a form of mindfulness meditation that can help to ground the mind in the present moment and promote relaxation.

Find a comfortable place to lie down, such as a bed or a mat. Make sure you are warm enough and that you have a comfortable support for your head.

Close your eyes and take a few deep breaths, focusing on the sensation of the breath as it enters and leaves your body. This can help to ground you in the present moment and bring your attention inward.

Begin to focus on your toes and the sensation of the toes on your feet. Notice any sensations of tingling, warmth, or pressure. Try to keep your focus on the toes for a few moments before moving on.

Slowly move your attention up the body,

focusing on each part for a few moments before moving on. You can focus on the soles of your feet, your ankles, your calves, your knees, and so on, until you reach the top of your head. As you focus on each part, try to stay present with any sensations that arise, without trying to change them.

If your mind wanders, gently redirect your attention back to the body. It's natural for the mind to wander, and this is not a sign of failure. Simply notice when your mind has wandered, and bring your attention back to the body.

Continue to focus on the body for as long as you like, allowing yourself to sink into a state of relaxation.

Body scan meditation can be a helpful tool for promoting relaxation and reducing stress and anxiety. It can also be a useful way to become more attuned to the sensations in your body, which can be helpful for managing chronic pain or other physical discomfort.

As with any meditation practice, it may take some time and effort to get the hang of it, but with regular practice, you may begin to see the benefits in your daily life.

Walking meditation

a type of meditation that involves focusing on the sensation of each step as you walk. It is another form of mindfulness meditation that can help to ground the mind in the present moment and promote a sense of calm and well-being.

Find a quiet place to walk, such as a park or a secluded path. Make sure you have enough space to walk in a straight line without obstructions.

Begin walking at a slow, leisurely pace. Pay attention to the sensation of each step as you walk. Notice the sensation of your feet touching the ground, the movement of your legs, and the sensation of your body moving through space.

As you walk, try to keep your focus on the sensation of the walk itself. You can repeat a mantra or phrase to yourself, such as "left foot, right foot," to help keep your focus on the present moment.

When your mind wanders (which it will), gently redirect your attention back to the sensation of the walk. It's natural for the mind to wander, and this is not a sign of failure. Simply notice when your mind has wandered, and bring your attention back to the present moment.

Continue to focus on the sensation of the walk for as long as you like, allowing yourself to sink into a state of mindfulness and relaxation.

Loving-kindness meditation

also known as "metta" meditation, is a type of meditation that involves cultivating feelings of love, kindness, and compassion towards oneself and others. It is based on the idea that all beings, including ourselves, have the capacity for love and that cultivating these positive emotions can bring about feelings of happiness and well-being.

Find a comfortable seated position with your back straight and your eyes closed. You can use a meditation cushion or sit on a chair with your feet planted firmly on the ground.

Take a few deep breaths and focus on the sensation of the breath as it enters and leaves your body. This can help to ground you in the present moment and bring your attention inward.

Bring to mind someone you love and care about deeply. It could be a family member, a close friend, or a beloved pet. As you think of this person, silently repeat the following phrases to yourself "May you be happy. May you be healthy. May you be safe. May you live with ease."

As you repeat these phrases, try to sincerely wish well-being for this person and visualize them surrounded by love and positivity.

Next, bring to mind someone you have neutral feelings towards, such as a coworker or a stranger. Again, silently repeat the phrases of loving-kindness to yourself "May you be happy. May you be healthy. May you be safe. May you live with ease.'

Again, try to sincerely wish well-being for this person and visualize them surrounded by love and positivity.

Finally, bring to mind someone you have difficulty with or hold resentment towards.

This could be someone who has caused you harm or someone with whom you have a strained relationship.

As challenging as it may be, try to repeat the phrases of loving-kindness to yourself "May you be happy. May you be healthy. May you be safe. May you live with ease."

It's important to note that this does not mean condoning any harm that may have been done, but rather recognizing the shared humanity of all beings and offering well-wishes for their well-being.

After you have directed loving-kindness towards these three individuals, you can expand the circle of love to include all beings. Silently repeat the phrases of loving-kindness to yourself "May all beings be happy. May all beings be healthy. May all beings be safe. May all beings live with ease."

Continue to focus on the phrases of loving-kindness for as long as you like, allowing the feelings of love and compassion to wash over you. When your mind wanders, gently redirect your attention back to the phrases.

loving-kindness meditation can be challenging at first, especially if you have difficulty feeling love towards yourself or others. However, with practice, it can help to cultivate feelings of compassion and connection, and can bring about a sense of peace and well-being.

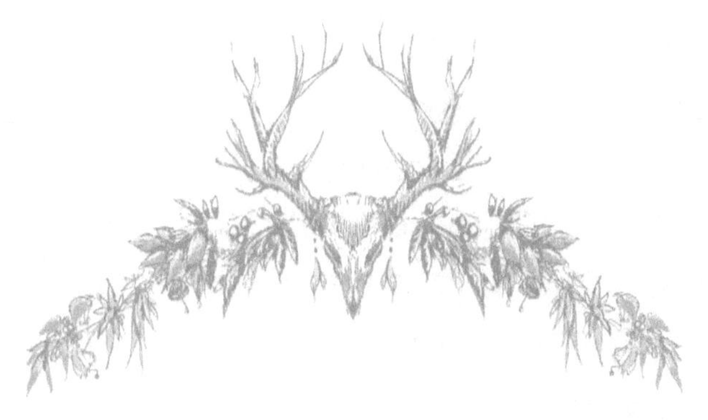

"*It does not matter how slowly you go as long as you do not stop.*"

- Confucius

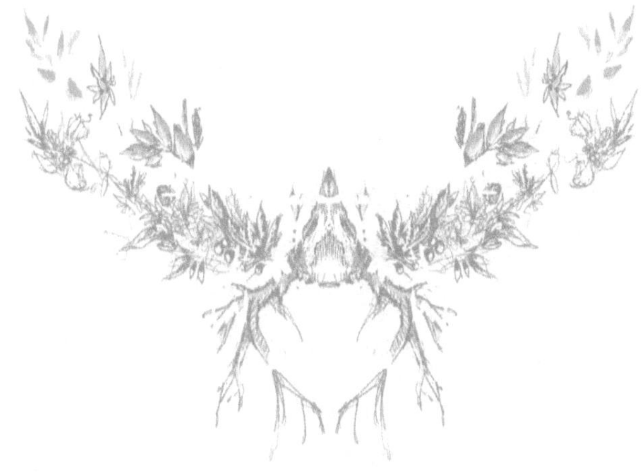

Breathing Exercise

A breathing exercise that may be helpful for you is the "4-7-8" technique, also known as "relaxing breath" or "the calming breath." This technique is simple to learn and can be done anywhere, at any time.

To perform the 4-7-8 technique, follow these steps Sit or lie down in a comfortable position, with your back straight and your hands on your lap.

Close your eyes and take a deep breath in through your nose, counting to four in your head.Hold your breath for a count of seven.

Exhale slowly through your mouth for a count of eight.

Repeat this cycle for several minutes, focusing on your breath and the counting.

The 4-7-8 technique is believed to help slow down the heart rate and calm the mind, which can be particularly beneficial for those with ADHD. It can also help to reduce anxiety, stress, and insomnia. It is recommended to practice it twice a day for at least two minutes each time, and to increase the duration gradually over time.

Stress Management techniques

Progressive Muscle Relaxation

Progressive Muscle Relaxation (PMR) is a technique that involves tensing and then relaxing different muscle groups in the body to help reduce tension and stress. The idea behind PMR is that by tensing and then relaxing the muscles, you can learn to recognize the feeling of muscle tension and relaxation, which can help you to relax more easily in other situations.

Here is a step-by-step guide to performing PMR

Find a quiet and comfortable place where you can sit or lie down. Starting with your feet, tense the muscles as tightly as you can for a count of 5-10 seconds.

Then, release the tension and feel the muscles relax.

Move on to the next muscle group, such as your calves and then your thighs, and repeat the process of tensing and relaxing.

Continue working your way up through the muscle groups of your body, including your stomach, back, chest, arms, hands, neck and face.

Once you have gone through all the muscle groups, spend a few minutes focusing on your breathing and allowing your body to fully relax.

Repeat the process as often as you like, aiming for at least once a day.

You can also try to do this by following an audio guide, or by using an app to guide you through the process.

It can take time and practice to learn how to relax your muscles and to get the most benefit from PMR, so try to be patient and consistent with the practice.

Guided imagery

This is a relaxation technique that involves using visualization and imagination to create a peaceful scene in the mind. The goal of guided imagery is to help a person to relax and feel more calm and peaceful.

Here is how to perform guided imagery

Find a quiet and comfortable place where you can sit or lie down. Close your eyes and take a few deep breaths.

Begin to imagine a peaceful scene in your mind. This can be a place you have been before, such as a beach or a forest, or it can be a place you have never been but would like to visit.

Imagine as many details as you can about the scene, such as the sound of the waves or the smell of the trees.

Imagine yourself in the scene and focus on how it makes you feel.

Continue to focus on the scene and let your mind wander.

If your mind begins to wander or if you start to feel distracted, gently bring your attention back to the peaceful scene.

Continue the visualization for as long as you like, aiming for at least 10 minutes.

It's important to note that it can take time and practice to get the most benefit from guided imagery, so it's important to be patient and consistent with the practice.

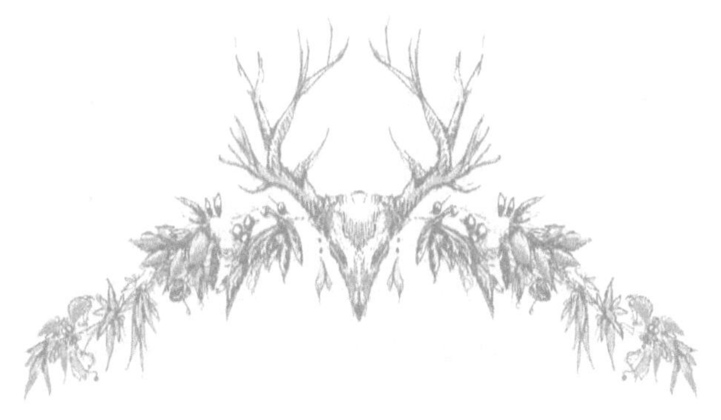

"The mind is everythin g;
what you think you become.

\- Buddha

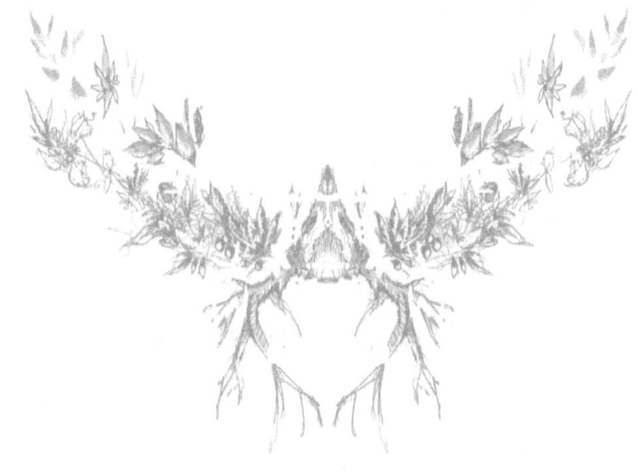

Music therapy

Music therapy is the use of music to improve a person's mental, physical, emotional, and/or social well-being.

The goal of music therapy is to help a person relax and feel more calm and peaceful.

How to use music therapy

Find a quiet and comfortable place where you can sit or lie down, ideally in a room with dim lighting and minimal distractions. Make sure you are wearing comfortable clothing and take a few deep breaths to help you relax.

Create a playlist of music that you find relaxing and that is appropriate for the setting. Some people may find classical music or nature sounds to be relaxing, while others may prefer soft, slow-paced songs.

Put on the music and focus on listening to it, paying attention to the melody, rhythm, and lyrics of the songs.

Close your eyes and let the music take you to a peaceful place in your mind.

As you listen to the music, focus on your breath and try to breathe deeply and slowly.

If your mind begins to wander or if you start to feel distracted, gently bring your attention back to the music.

Use the music as a focal point to help you relax and let go of any stress or tension you may be feeling.

Continue to listen to the music for as long as you like, aiming for at least 10-15 minutes.

After you finish the listening session, take a moment to reflect on how you feel and make note of it.

The key to music therapy is to find music that you enjoy and that helps you to relax. It's also good to be consistent with the practice, listening to music regularly and experimenting with different types of music to find what works best for you.

Cognitive Behavioral Therapy

Cognitive Behavioral Therapy (CBT) is a form of therapy that focuses on changing negative thought patterns and behaviors. It can be a useful tool for people with ADHD to learn how to better manage their symptoms and improve their overall functioning.

Understand the basic principles of CBT

CBT is based on the idea that our thoughts, feelings, and behaviors are interconnected, and that changing one aspect of this triangle can have a positive impact on the other two.

Identify negative thoughts and patterns.

Start by identifying negative thoughts and patterns that may be contributing to your symptoms of ADHD. Examples may include thoughts like "I can't focus," "I'm lazy," or "I'm not good enough." Challenge negative thoughts Once you have identified a negative thought, challenge it by asking yourself questions like "Is this thought really true?" or "Is there any evidence to support or refute this thought?"

Replace negative thoughts with positive ones

Once you have challenged a negative thought, try to replace it with a more positive or realistic one. For example, instead of thinking "I can't focus," try thinking "I may have difficulty focusing sometimes, but I can work on strategies to improve my attention."

Identify triggers

Identify situations or activities that trigger your symptoms of ADHD. Examples may include things like working on long-term projects, studying for exams, or attending meetings.

Develop coping strategies

Once you have identified triggers, develop coping strategies to help you manage your symptoms in those situations. Examples may include things like breaking down large tasks into smaller, more manageable chunks, using a planner or calendar to stay organized, or taking regular breaks to move around and refocus.

Practice, practice, practice

CBT is an ongoing process and requires consistent practice to be effective. Make sure to schedule regular "check-ins" with yourself to review your progress, and be patient with yourself as you work to develop new habits and thought patterns.

CBT requires a certain level of self-awareness and willingness to change. It's also important to work with a therapist that has experience working with ADHD patients. This therapy can help you to learn how to manage your symptoms and improve your overall functioning.

Social skills training

Social skills training is a form of therapy that helps individuals with ADHD improve their social interactions and relationships.

It can be beneficial for those who have difficulty with communication, understanding social cues, and maintaining friendships. Here's a guide to use social skills training therapy for ADHD.

Understand the basics

Social skills training therapy is based on the idea that Social interactions and relationships can be learned and improved through practice and guidance.

Identify areas of difficulty

Identify areas where you are struggling in your social interactions and relationships, such as initiating conversations, understanding social cues, or maintaining friendships.

Learn specific social skills

Learn specific social skills such as active listening, perspective taking, and understanding and expressing emotions.

Practice social skills

Practice the social skills you have learned in a safe and controlled environment, such as through role-playing exercises, group therapy, or video feedback sessions with a therapist.

Use real-life situations

Practice the skills in real-life situations by setting up social opportunities with friends or family members, or by volunteering in a community setting.

Get feedback

Get feedback from others on your social interactions and relationships by asking for honest feedback from friends or family members or by receiving feedback from a therapist or counselor. Reflect on progress Reflect on your progress and identify areas where you still need to improve. With practice this will give you tools and strategies you can use in your daily life to better interact with friends, family and colleges.

Difficulties with sleep

Being well rested is the basis when working with yourself, which makes it so annoying that people with ADHD often have difficulties with sleep. Here are some points you can try which can better your chances of falling asleep faster.

Create a bedtime routine

Establishing a consistent bedtime routine can help to signal to the body that it's time to wind down and prepare for sleep. This might include activities such as taking a warm bath, reading a book, or practicing relaxation techniques.

Reduce stimulants

Caffeine, nicotine, and other stimulants can interfere with sleep and should be avoided in the hours leading up to bedtime. It can also be helpful to limit screen time before bed, as the blue light emitted by screens can disrupt the body's natural sleep-wake cycle.

Practice relaxation techniques

Techniques such as deep breathing, progressive muscle relaxation, or guided imagery can help to calm the mind and promote relaxation. These techniques can be practiced in bed or in the hours leading up to bedtime.

Establish a sleep-friendly environment

Creating a comfortable, cool, and dark sleep environment can help to promote sleep. This might include using a comfortable mattress and pillows, keeping the room at a comfortable temperature, and using blackout curtains or an eye mask to block out light.

Consider using sleep aids

If sleep difficulties persist despite trying these techniques, it may be helpful to speak with a healthcare provider about the use of sleep aids. There are several options available, including over-the-counter and prescription medications, as well as non-pharmacological options such as white noise machines or weighted blankets.

Final Words

Living with ADHD can be challenging.

We understand that the symptoms of ADHD can make it difficult to manage time and complete tasks effectively, and that it can affect your daily life in many ways.

Remember that you are not defined by your condition and that you have the strength and capability to manage your life.

ADHD can be isolating and it can be hard to find people who understand what you're going through. But remember that you are not alone, and there is help and support available. Reach out to your family and friends, join a support group, or talk to a therapist or counselor who can provide you with the support you need.

It's also important to remember that you are not to blame for your condition, and that it is not a sign of weakness or laziness. ADHD is a real and legitimate condition, and it's important to take care of yourself and manage your symptoms as best as you can.

We also want to remind you that it's okay to ask for help. Many people with ADHD struggle with feeling overwhelmed, and remember that it's okay to ask for help when you need it.

Don't be afraid to ask for help with tasks or projects, or to ask for accommodation.

Lastly, we want to remind you that you are capable of achieving great things, and don't let ADHD define who you are.

With the right tools and mindset, you can build resilience and find success in your daily life. Be kind to yourself, and celebrate your progress along the way.

Find the right approach for you, and that may require some trial and error, but with determination and perseverance, you can overcome any obstacle that comes your way.

You have the power to take control of your life and live it to the fullest. So don't give up, keep going and know that you are not alone.

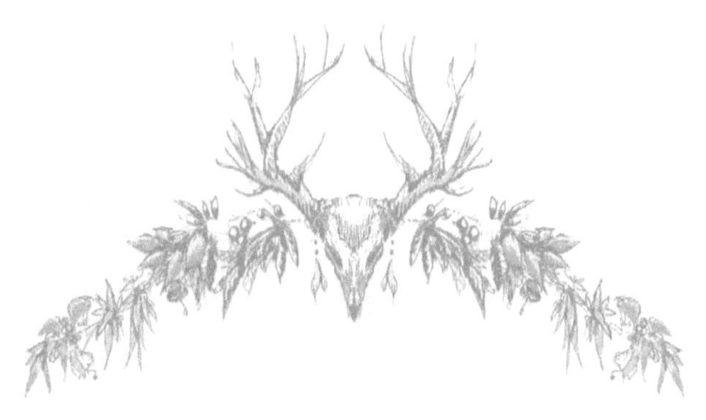

*"You are not weak for struggling;
you are strong for surviving"*

-Oak & Leaf

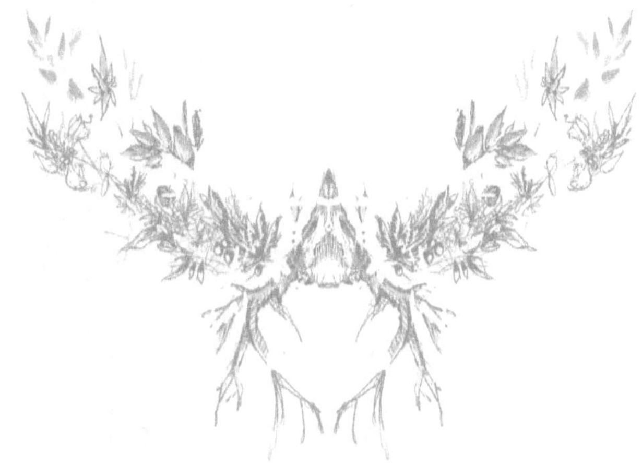